THE ALASKAPOX SCARE

Prevention, Awareness, and the Fight for a Cure for a Newly Identified Viral Disease

Readers Realm

Disclaimer

The information in this book is provided for general informational purposes only. While every effort has been made to ensure the accuracy and completeness of the content, the author and publisher assume no responsibility for errors, inaccuracies, or omissions. The author and publisher shall have no liability to any person or entity with respect to any loss or damage caused or alleged to be caused directly or indirectly by the information contained in this book.

Table of Contents

INTRODUCTION

In the intricate web of our planet's ecosystems, the emergence of infectious diseases poses a constant challenge to both human and animal populations. Among these threats looms Alaskapox, a newly identified viral disease that has captured global attention. With its origins rooted in the wilderness of Alaska, Alaskapox serves as a stark reminder of the interconnectedness between wildlife health and human well-being. This book delves into the fascinating story of Alaskapox, tracing its discovery, clinical manifestations, and societal implications. From the forests of the Kenai Peninsula to the laboratories of public health agencies, we embark on a journey to understand the complexities of this enigmatic virus and the efforts underway to combat its spread. Through exploration of wildlife ecology, public health response strategies, and lessons learned from past outbreaks, we aim to shed light on the broader challenges posed by emerging infectious diseases and the imperative of proactive measures in safeguarding global health security.

Chapter 1

The Origins of Alaskapox

The discovery of Alaskapox is a testament to the vigilance of public health officials and the advancements in diagnostic technology. In 2015, health authorities in Fairbanks, Alaska, were alerted to a perplexing case involving a patient exhibiting symptoms consistent with a viral infection. The patient presented with a fever, rash, and lymphadenopathy, prompting healthcare providers to conduct thorough diagnostic tests. Upon isolating the causative agent from the patient's blood samples, researchers identified a previously unknown virus, which would later be designated as Alaskapox. This groundbreaking discovery sparked a flurry of scientific inquiry as experts sought to understand the origins and implications of this novel pathogen.

Classification within the Orthopox Group

Alaskapox, like its counterparts in the Orthopox genus, shares genetic similarities with other members of the family, including smallpox and monkeypox. However, distinct genomic characteristics distinguish Alaskapox as a separate species within this group. Through genome sequencing and comparative analysis, researchers have elucidated the genetic makeup of Alaskapox, shedding light on its evolutionary history and phylogenetic relationships. This classification not only aids in understanding the biology of the virus but also informs efforts to develop targeted diagnostic assays and therapeutic interventions.

Initial Cases and Spread in Alaska

Following its initial identification in Fairbanks, Alaskapox rapidly disseminated throughout Alaska, fueled by interactions between humans and wildlife. The first cases predominantly occurred in rural and semi-rural areas, where individuals engaged in activities that increased their exposure to wildlife habitats. Hunters, trappers, and outdoor enthusiasts were among the first to report symptoms suggestive of Alaskapox, indicating zoonotic transmission from infected animals to humans. As the virus continued to circulate within wildlife populations, additional cases emerged in other regions of the state, including the Kenai Peninsula and Anchorage. The geographical spread of Alaskapox underscored the need for comprehensive surveillance and control measures to prevent further transmission and mitigate the impact on public health.

Challenges in Detection and Diagnosis

Despite advances in diagnostic techniques, the identification of Alaskapox presents unique challenges due to its rarity and similarity to other orthopoxviruses. Clinical manifestations of Alaskapox often overlap with those of other viral illnesses, complicating diagnosis and delaying appropriate treatment. Moreover, limited access to specialized laboratory facilities and trained personnel in remote areas of Alaska can impede timely detection of cases, exacerbating the risk of secondary transmission. Addressing these challenges requires coordinated efforts to enhance surveillance capabilities, improve access to diagnostic resources, and raise awareness among healthcare providers about the clinical features of Alaskapox.

Future Directions in Research

As the scientific community continues to unravel the complexities of Alaskapox, several avenues for future research emerge. Understanding the ecological factors driving virus transmission between wildlife and humans is paramount for predicting and preventing future outbreaks. Additionally, efforts to develop effective vaccines and antiviral therapies against Alaskapox remain ongoing, with promising candidates undergoing preclinical evaluation. Collaborative initiatives between government agencies, academic institutions, and international partners are essential for advancing our knowledge of Alaskapox and mitigating its impact on public health.

Chapter 2

Clinical Manifestations and Epidemiology

Alaskapox, a member of the orthopoxvirus family, presents with a spectrum of symptoms in infected individuals, with severity ranging from mild to severe. Typically, the onset of symptoms occurs within a week of exposure to the virus. Initially, patients may experience non-specific flu-like symptoms, including fever, fatigue, headache, and muscle aches. These early symptoms can often be mistaken for common viral infections, making early diagnosis challenging.

As the disease progresses, characteristic skin lesions develop, usually beginning as small, red bumps that gradually evolve into fluid-filled vesicles. These vesicles eventually crust over and form scabs, which can be itchy and painful. The lesions can appear anywhere on the body but are commonly found in areas where the skin has been damaged or irritated, such as the hands, face, and groin.

In immunocompromised individuals, such as those undergoing chemotherapy or organ transplant recipients, Alaskapox infections can lead to more severe complications. These may include pneumonia, encephalitis (inflammation of the brain), or systemic infection, which can be life-threatening if not promptly treated. Additionally, elderly individuals and those with underlying health conditions are at increased risk of experiencing severe disease outcomes.

Early recognition of symptoms and prompt medical evaluation are crucial for effectively managing Alaskapox cases and preventing severe outcomes. Healthcare providers should maintain a high index of suspicion for Alaskapox, especially in individuals with a history of exposure to wildlife or living in areas where the virus is known to circulate.

Epidemiological Characteristics and Transmission Dynamics

Understanding the epidemiology of Alaskapox is essential for controlling its spread and preventing further outbreaks. Epidemiological studies have revealed several key characteristics of the virus, including its mode of transmission and patterns of spread within human populations.

Alaskapox primarily spreads through direct contact with infected animals or their bodily fluids, such as saliva or respiratory secretions. Human-to-human transmission is rare but can occur through close contact with infected individuals or contaminated objects. Additionally, the virus can survive on surfaces for extended periods, increasing the risk of transmission through fomites.

Certain populations are at increased risk of Alaskapox infection, including individuals with occupational exposure to wildlife, such as hunters, trappers, or wildlife biologists. Living in or near areas with high populations of small mammals, such as voles or squirrels, also increases the risk of exposure to the virus.

To control the spread of Alaskapox, public health officials employ various strategies, including surveillance, contact tracing, and isolation of infected individuals. Vaccination may play a role in preventing future outbreaks, although no specific vaccine for Alaskapox currently exists. Continued research into the epidemiology and transmission dynamics of the virus is essential for informing public health policies and guiding effective disease control measures.

Chapter 3

Wildlife Ecology and Disease Transmission

Small mammals are integral components of ecosystems, serving diverse ecological functions and playing vital roles in maintaining ecosystem balance. However, they also serve as reservoirs and vectors for a wide array of zoonotic pathogens, including viruses, bacteria, and parasites. Among these pathogens is the Alaskapox virus, a newly identified orthopoxvirus that has been linked to small mammal populations in Alaska.

The lifecycle of Alaskapox involves transmission between small mammals, typically through direct contact or exposure to contaminated materials such as feces or urine. While the virus does not usually cause severe illness in these animals, they can serve as asymptomatic carriers, shedding the virus into the environment and facilitating its transmission to other susceptible hosts, including humans.

Voles, in particular, have been implicated as significant carriers of the Alaskapox virus due to their high population densities and close association with human settlements. These small rodents are highly adaptable and can thrive in a variety of habitats, ranging from grasslands and forests to urban areas. Their abundance and ecological flexibility make them efficient vectors for disease transmission, facilitating the spread of Alaskapox within and beyond their native range.

The role of small mammals in zoonotic disease transmission underscores the importance of understanding their ecology and behavior in order to mitigate the risk of disease outbreaks. Research efforts focused on characterizing the interactions between small mammals, pathogens, and the environment can provide valuable insights into the dynamics of disease transmission and inform strategies for disease surveillance and control.

Moreover, the identification of Alaskapox in small mammal populations highlights the need for ongoing monitoring and surveillance of wildlife diseases, particularly in regions where human-wildlife interactions are prevalent. By studying the ecology of small mammals and their role in disease transmission, scientists can develop targeted interventions aimed at reducing the transmission of zoonotic pathogens and protecting human and animal health.

Impact of Human Activities on Wildlife Habitats

Human activities exert significant pressures on wildlife habitats, leading to habitat loss, fragmentation, and degradation. These anthropogenic changes to natural ecosystems can have profound impacts on wildlife populations and their interactions with pathogens, influencing the dynamics of disease transmission and emergence.

Deforestation, urbanization, agricultural expansion, and infrastructure development are among the primary drivers of habitat destruction worldwide. These activities result in the loss and degradation of wildlife habitats, forcing animals into closer proximity to human settlements and activities. As a result, the likelihood of zoonotic spillover events increases, as animals come into contact with humans and domestic animals, facilitating the transmission of pathogens like the Alaskapox virus.

In Alaska, where Alaskapox was first identified, human activities such as logging, mining, and recreational pursuits have encroached upon wilderness areas, altering the natural landscape and disrupting wildlife habitats. These changes can influence the distribution and behavior of small mammals, affecting the dynamics of disease transmission in complex ways.

Additionally, climate change poses significant challenges to wildlife habitats and disease transmission dynamics. Rising temperatures, altered precipitation patterns, and habitat modifications associated with climate change can impact the distribution and abundance of wildlife species, potentially altering the transmission dynamics of zoonotic diseases like Alaskapox. As habitats shift and ecosystems undergo transformations, the risk of disease emergence and spread may increase, necessitating adaptive management strategies to mitigate these risks.

Addressing the impact of human activities on wildlife habitats and disease transmission requires a multifaceted approach that integrates conservation, land-use planning, and public health initiatives. Protecting and restoring natural ecosystems, promoting sustainable land management practices, and fostering coexistence between humans and wildlife are essential components of efforts to mitigate the risk of zoonotic disease transmission while preserving biodiversity and ecosystem health. By recognizing the interconnectedness of human health, wildlife ecology, and environmental conservation, we can work towards sustainable solutions that safeguard both human and animal populations from the threat of emerging infectious diseases like Alaskapox.

Chapter 4

Public Health Response and Preparedness

In the wake of emerging infectious diseases like Alaskapox, public health agencies are tasked with mounting a comprehensive response to mitigate the spread of the virus and protect vulnerable populations. This chapter delves into the multifaceted strategies employed by public health authorities, encompassing surveillance and diagnostic capabilities, proactive measures for disease prevention and control, and the critical role of vaccination and immunization in curtailing the impact of Alaskapox on human health.

Surveillance and Diagnostic Capabilities

Surveillance serves as the cornerstone of early detection and response efforts, enabling public health officials to monitor trends in disease incidence and identify potential outbreaks. For Alaskapox, surveillance efforts extend beyond human populations to encompass wildlife species known to harbor the virus, such as voles and other small mammals. Collaborative partnerships between healthcare providers, laboratories, and wildlife agencies facilitate data sharing and enhance the efficiency of surveillance systems.

Enhancing diagnostic capabilities is paramount for promptly identifying cases of

Alaskapox and implementing appropriate control measures. Current diagnostic methods primarily rely on polymerase chain reaction (PCR) assays to detect viral genetic material in patient samples, such as blood or tissue specimens. However, the development of rapid diagnostic tests capable of detecting viral antigens or antibodies could significantly improve diagnostic efficiency and enable more timely interventions.

In addition to traditional surveillance methods, innovative approaches such as syndromic surveillance and digital disease detection systems hold promise for enhancing early detection of Alaskapox outbreaks. By leveraging data from various sources, including healthcare records, social media, and environmental sensors, these systems can detect patterns indicative of disease transmission and facilitate targeted response efforts.

Proactive Measures for Disease Prevention and Control

Preventing the spread of Alaskapox necessitates a multi-faceted approach that encompasses both individual and community-level interventions. Public health agencies collaborate with community stakeholders to implement strategies aimed at reducing human-wildlife contact, such as wildlife management programs and public education campaigns promoting safe handling practices. Vector control measures targeting disease-carrying animals, such as rodents, may also be employed to minimize the risk of transmission to humans.

Community engagement plays a pivotal role in fostering adherence to preventive measures and promoting behavior change. Public health campaigns leverage various communication channels, including traditional media, social media, and community outreach events, to disseminate information about Alaskapox and encourage adoption of recommended preventive measures. By empowering communities to take ownership of their health and well-being, public health agencies can enhance the effectiveness of disease prevention efforts and foster resilience against Alaskapox and other emerging infectious diseases.

Importance of Vaccination and Immunization

Vaccination and immunization represent indispensable tools in the arsenal of infectious disease prevention. While no vaccine currently exists for Alaskapox, ongoing research efforts seek to develop candidate vaccines capable of eliciting protective immune responses against the virus. Parallel efforts may focus on immunization against related orthopoxviruses, such as smallpox and monkeypox, which could provide cross-protection against Alaskapox. Furthermore, maintaining high vaccination coverage rates for preventable diseases reduces the overall burden on healthcare systems and helps mitigate the risk of co-infections with Alaskapox.

Public health agencies play a central role in promoting vaccination and immunization through targeted outreach efforts and vaccine distribution programs. Robust immunization registries enable healthcare providers to track vaccine coverage rates and identify areas requiring additional vaccination efforts. By prioritizing vaccination research and development and strengthening immunization infrastructure, public health officials can enhance resilience against Alaskapox and other emerging infectious diseases.

In conclusion, a multifaceted approach to public health response and preparedness is essential for effectively addressing the threat of Alaskapox. By bolstering surveillance and diagnostic capabilities, implementing proactive measures for disease prevention and control, and prioritizing vaccination and immunization efforts, public health agencies can mitigate the impact of Alaskapox on human health and safeguard communities against future outbreaks.

Chapter 5

Societal Implications and Policy Considerations

The emergence of Alaskapox has far-reaching implications beyond the realm of public health. From economic disruptions to social upheavals, the impact of this novel viral disease reverberates across various sectors of society.

Economically, Alaskapox poses significant challenges to affected communities. The outbreak can disrupt local economies, particularly in regions reliant on outdoor tourism and recreational activities. With concerns over disease transmission, tourism may decline, leading to revenue losses for businesses and individuals dependent on this industry. Moreover, healthcare costs associated with diagnosing and treating Alaskapox cases can strain already burdened healthcare systems, particularly in rural areas with limited access to medical resources.

Socially, the fear and uncertainty surrounding Alaskapox can exacerbate existing tensions within communities. Stigma and discrimination against individuals perceived to be at risk or infected with the virus can lead to social isolation and marginalization. Furthermore, misinformation and rumors circulating about Alaskapox can sow seeds of distrust and division among community members, hindering effective disease control efforts.

Psychologically, the psychological toll of living in the midst of an outbreak cannot be underestimated. Anxiety, fear, and stress permeate the lives of individuals and families grappling with the threat of Alaskapox. Concerns over personal safety, livelihoods, and the well-being of loved ones weigh heavily on the minds of those affected by the disease. Additionally, the psychological impact of witnessing severe illness and death, particularly among vulnerable populations, can leave lasting scars on individuals and communities.

In light of these economic, social, and psychological impacts, policymakers must adopt a holistic approach to addressing the challenges posed by Alaskapox. Efforts to mitigate the consequences of the outbreak must go beyond medical interventions and encompass measures to support affected communities, promote social cohesion, and safeguard mental health.

Policy Considerations for Disease Control and Prevention

Effective disease control and prevention strategies are essential for containing the spread of Alaskapox and minimizing its impact on public health. Policymakers play a crucial role in formulating and implementing policies that address the various facets of the outbreak, from surveillance and diagnosis to treatment and containment.

One key policy consideration is the establishment of robust surveillance systems to monitor the spread of Alaskapox and identify emerging hotspots of transmission. Enhanced surveillance capabilities, including the use of advanced diagnostic technologies and data analytics, can provide early warning signs of outbreaks and inform targeted intervention efforts.

Another policy consideration is the implementation of preventive measures to reduce the risk of Alaskapox transmission within communities. This may include promoting personal hygiene practices, such as handwashing and respiratory etiquette, and implementing social distancing measures to minimize close contact between individuals.

Furthermore, policymakers must prioritize the allocation of resources to support healthcare infrastructure and capacity-building initiatives in regions affected by Alaskapox. This may involve investing in medical facilities, training healthcare workers, and stockpiling essential medical supplies and equipment to ensure prompt and effective response to outbreaks.

Additionally, policies aimed at promoting vaccination and immunization coverage are essential for preventing future outbreaks of Alaskapox. Vaccination campaigns targeting high-risk populations, such as individuals with compromised immune systems or those living in endemic regions, can help build herd immunity and reduce the overall burden of the disease.

In formulating disease control and prevention policies, policymakers must also consider ethical and equity considerations, ensuring that interventions are equitable, transparent, and respectful of individual rights and freedoms.

Community Engagement and Risk Communication

Effective risk communication and community engagement are critical components of successful disease control and prevention efforts. Engaging with communities affected by Alaskapox fosters trust, promotes cooperation, and empowers individuals to take proactive measures to protect themselves and their loved ones.

One key aspect of community engagement is providing accurate and timely information about Alaskapox, including its transmission dynamics, symptoms, and prevention strategies. Transparent communication helps dispel rumors and misinformation, empowering individuals to make informed decisions about their health and safety.

Furthermore, community engagement efforts should involve collaboration with local leaders, community organizations, and grassroots networks to reach diverse populations and address unique cultural and linguistic needs. Tailoring messages to resonate with specific community values, beliefs, and practices enhances the effectiveness of risk communication efforts and promotes greater adherence to preventive measures.

Moreover, community engagement should not be limited to information dissemination but should also involve meaningful dialogue and participation in decision-making processes. Soliciting feedback from community members, incorporating local knowledge and expertise, and fostering partnerships with community stakeholders facilitate the co-creation of solutions that are contextually relevant and culturally sensitive.

By prioritizing community engagement and risk communication, policymakers can build trust, strengthen social cohesion, and mobilize collective action to combat the spread of Alaskapox. Empowering communities to take ownership of their health and well-being is essential for fostering resilience and ensuring effective disease control and prevention in the face of emerging infectious diseases.

Economic impacts of Alaskapox include disruptions in various sectors such as tourism, healthcare, and local businesses.

Tourism-dependent areas may experience a decline in visitors due to fear of disease transmission, leading to revenue losses and economic strain for businesses reliant on tourism. Additionally, healthcare systems may face increased costs associated with diagnosing and treating Alaskapox cases, particularly in rural areas with limited access to medical resources. Social impacts include stigma and discrimination against individuals perceived to be at risk or infected with the virus. Misinformation and rumors circulating about Alaskapox can further exacerbate social tensions and hinder effective disease control efforts. Psychological impacts encompass the emotional toll of living in the midst of an outbreak, including anxiety, fear, and stress. Concerns over personal safety, livelihoods, and the well-being of loved ones can take a significant toll on mental health, particularly among vulnerable populations.

Policy considerations for disease control and prevention include establishing robust surveillance systems to monitor the spread of Alaskapox and identify emerging hotspots of transmission. Enhanced surveillance capabilities, including advanced diagnostic technologies and data analytics, can provide early warning signs of outbreaks and inform targeted intervention efforts. Preventive measures may include promoting personal hygiene practices, implementing social distancing measures, and prioritizing vaccination and immunization campaigns. Furthermore, policymakers must allocate resources to support healthcare infrastructure and capacity-building initiatives in regions affected by Alaskapox, ensuring prompt and effective response to outbreaks. Ethical and equity considerations are also paramount in policy formulation, ensuring interventions are equitable, transparent, and respectful of individual rights and freedoms.

Community engagement and risk communication efforts are crucial for building trust, promoting cooperation, and empowering individuals to take proactive measures to protect themselves and their communities. Providing accurate and timely information about Alaskapox, tailored to resonate with specific community values and beliefs, helps dispel rumors and misinformation, empowering individuals to make informed decisions about their health and safety. Collaborating with local leaders, organizations, and grassroots networks facilitates the co-creation of solutions that are contextually relevant and culturally sensitive. By prioritizing community engagement and risk communication, policymakers can foster resilience and mobilize collective action to combat the spread of Alaskapox, ensuring effective disease control and prevention in the face of emerging infectious diseases.

Chapter 6

Prevention and Mitigation Strategies

Emerging infectious diseases like Alaskapox present significant challenges to public health authorities, healthcare providers, and communities. In this chapter, we delve into a comprehensive exploration of various prevention and mitigation strategies aimed at reducing the risk of Alaskapox transmission and minimizing its impact on human and animal populations.

Personal Protective Measures to Reduce Risk of Infection

Personal protective measures play a pivotal role in preventing the spread of infectious diseases like Alaskapox. Individuals can take proactive steps to reduce their risk of infection and protect themselves and others from the virus.

Hand Hygiene

Rigorous hand hygiene practices are foundational in preventing the transmission of Alaskapox. Regular handwashing with soap and water for at least 20 seconds, especially after being in public places or touching potentially contaminated surfaces, is highly recommended. Hand sanitizers containing at least 60% alcohol can also serve as an effective alternative when soap and water are not readily available.

Avoiding Close Contact

The virus primarily spreads through respiratory droplets produced when an infected person coughs, sneezes, or talks. Thus, maintaining physical distance from individuals who are sick or displaying symptoms of Alaskapox is crucial. Adhering to social distancing guidelines, particularly in crowded settings or enclosed spaces, can significantly reduce the risk of transmission.

Wearing Protective Clothing

When venturing into areas where Alaskapox transmission may occur, such as forests or wooded areas, wearing protective clothing can provide an additional layer of defense.

Long sleeves, pants, and gloves can act as barriers, minimizing direct contact with infected animals or their habitats.

Avoiding Wildlife Contact

Given the zoonotic nature of Alaskapox, minimizing contact with wildlife, particularly small mammals like voles and squirrels, is essential. Individuals should refrain from handling or feeding wild animals and should keep pets away from potentially infected areas to mitigate the risk of transmission.

Proper Wound Care

In cases where individuals may have been exposed to Alaskapox, proper wound care is imperative to prevent secondary infections and complications. Any cuts, scratches, or abrasions should be promptly cleaned and covered with sterile dressings to prevent contamination and facilitate healing.

Face Masks

While face masks may not be necessary for routine activities, they can be beneficial in situations where maintaining physical distancing is challenging. Wearing a face mask, particularly in crowded public spaces or during close contact with individuals who may be infected with Alaskapox, can provide an additional layer of protection for both the wearer and those around them.

By diligently adopting these personal protective measures, individuals can significantly reduce their risk of Alaskapox infection and contribute to community-wide efforts to control the spread of the virus.

Environmental Management Techniques to Minimize Disease Spread

In addition to personal protective measures, environmental management techniques play a pivotal role in minimizing the spread of Alaskapox and reducing the risk of transmission in natural habitats. These techniques focus on modifying the environment to create barriers to disease transmission and reduce contact between susceptible hosts and the virus.

Habitat Modification

Modifying wildlife habitats to reduce the density of small mammal populations can help limit the spread of Alaskapox. This may involve removing or altering habitat features that attract small mammals, such as dense vegetation or food sources. By disrupting the ecological conditions that facilitate disease transmission, habitat modification strategies can effectively mitigate the risk of Alaskapox transmission in natural ecosystems.

Vector Control

Controlling the populations of vectors that may transmit Alaskapox, such as ticks or fleas, is another crucial component of environmental management. Vector control measures, including the use of insecticide treatments or environmental modifications to reduce vector breeding sites, can help prevent the spread of the virus to humans and other animals. By targeting the vectors responsible for Alaskapox transmission, public health authorities can effectively disrupt the disease cycle and reduce the risk of human infection.

Surveillance and Monitoring

Regular surveillance and monitoring of wildlife populations are essential for detecting and tracking the spread of Alaskapox in natural habitats. By conducting targeted surveillance efforts and monitoring changes in disease prevalence and distribution, public health authorities can identify areas where Alaskapox transmission is occurring and implement timely control measures. Surveillance data can also inform the development of predictive models to anticipate future outbreaks and guide proactive interventions to prevent further spread of the virus.

Public Education and Outreach

Educating the public about the risks of Alaskapox and the importance of environmental management techniques is critical for fostering community engagement and participation in disease prevention efforts. Public education and outreach initiatives can include workshops, informational materials, and community events aimed at raising awareness about Alaskapox transmission dynamics and promoting behavioral changes to reduce the risk of infection. By empowering communities with knowledge and resources, public health authorities can mobilize collective action to protect human and animal populations from the threat of Alaskapox.

By implementing these environmental management techniques, communities can reduce the risk of Alaskapox transmission in natural habitats and mitigate the impact of the virus on human and animal populations.

Role of Healthcare Providers in Educating and Empowering Communities

Healthcare providers play a pivotal role in educating and empowering communities to prevent and mitigate the spread of Alaskapox. As trusted sources of information and guidance, healthcare providers have a unique opportunity to disseminate accurate information about

Alaskapox transmission, prevention, and treatment. Key aspects of the role of healthcare providers include:

Patient Education

Healthcare providers can play a crucial role in educating patients about the signs and symptoms of Alaskapox, as well as the importance of seeking medical care promptly if they suspect they may have been exposed to the virus. This includes providing information about the risks of Alaskapox transmission and the steps individuals can take to protect themselves and their families. By empowering patients with knowledge about Alaskapox prevention and control measures, healthcare providers can enhance awareness and promote proactive health-seeking behaviors.

Community Outreach

Healthcare providers can engage in community outreach efforts to raise awareness about Alaskapox and promote preventive measures among at-risk populations. This may involve participating in community events, giving presentations at local schools or community centers, and collaborating with public health authorities to disseminate information about Alaskapox transmission dynamics and prevention strategies. By leveraging their expertise and credibility within the community, healthcare providers can effectively reach diverse audiences and foster positive health outcomes.

Clinical Management

Healthcare providers play a crucial role in the clinical management of Alaskapox cases, including diagnosis, treatment, and follow-up care. This may involve conducting diagnostic tests, prescribing medications to alleviate symptoms, and monitoring patients for complications. By providing timely and appropriate medical care to individuals affected by Alaskapox, healthcare providers can mitigate the severity of illness and reduce the risk of complications. Additionally, healthcare providers can offer supportive care and counseling to patients and their families, addressing their concerns and promoting resilience in the face of adversity.

Advocacy and Policy Development

Healthcare providers can advocate for policies and interventions aimed at preventing and controlling Alaskapox at the local, regional, and national levels. This may include supporting funding for research, public health initiatives, and infrastructure improvements to enhance disease surveillance and response capabilities. By leveraging their expertise and influence, healthcare providers can contribute to the development and implementation of evidence-based strategies to combat Alaskapox and protect public health. Additionally, healthcare providers can collaborate with policymakers and stakeholders to address broader social determinants of health that may contribute to the spread of Alaskapox, such as access to healthcare, socioeconomic disparities, and environmental factors.

Mental Health Support

In addition to medical care, healthcare providers can offer mental health support to individuals and communities affected by Alaskapox. The fear and uncertainty surrounding the virus can take a toll on mental well-being, leading to anxiety, depression, and other psychological distress. Healthcare providers can provide psychoeducation about coping strategies, stress management techniques, and resources for accessing mental health services. By addressing the emotional and psychological needs of patients and their families, healthcare providers can promote resilience and facilitate recovery from the impacts of Alaskapox.

By actively engaging with patients and communities, healthcare providers can play a vital role in educating and empowering individuals to take proactive measures to prevent Alaskapox transmission and mitigate its impact on public health. Through patient education, community outreach, clinical management, advocacy, and mental health support, healthcare providers can contribute to comprehensive efforts to control the spread of Alaskapox and protect the well-being of populations at risk.

In this chapter, we have provided a detailed exploration of prevention and mitigation strategies for managing Alaskapox, including personal protective measures, environmental management techniques, and the critical role of healthcare providers in educating and empowering communities. By implementing these strategies in a coordinated and collaborative manner, we can reduce the impact of Alaskapox on human and animal populations and safeguard public health.

Chapter 7

Case Studies and Best Practices

In this chapter, we delve into case studies of successful disease prevention and control efforts, focusing on instances where proactive measures effectively mitigated the spread of infectious diseases. By examining these case studies, we can identify key strategies and best practices that have proven to be effective in containing outbreaks and reducing morbidity and mortality rates.

Case Study 1: Smallpox Eradication Program

One of the most notable success stories in the history of disease prevention is the global eradication of smallpox. Smallpox, caused by the variola virus, was a devastating infectious disease that plagued humanity for centuries, resulting in millions of deaths worldwide. However, through a coordinated effort led by the World Health Organization (WHO), smallpox was successfully eradicated, and the last known natural case occurred in 1977. The eradication campaign employed a combination of vaccination, surveillance, and containment strategies. Mass vaccination campaigns targeted vulnerable populations, while intensive surveillance efforts tracked down and isolated cases to prevent further spread. Additionally, the establishment of a global network of laboratories facilitated rapid diagnosis and response. This monumental achievement serves as a testament to the power of international collaboration and concerted public health interventions in combatting infectious diseases.

Case Study 2: Ebola Outbreak Response in West Africa

The Ebola virus outbreak that ravaged West Africa between 2014 and 2016 underscored the urgent need for effective response strategies to emerging infectious diseases. Ebola virus disease (EVD) is a highly lethal viral hemorrhagic fever with a case fatality rate of up to 90%. The outbreak, which primarily affected Guinea, Liberia, and Sierra Leone, resulted in over 28,000 reported cases and more than 11,000 deaths. However, despite the unprecedented scale of the epidemic, concerted efforts by local and international health organizations eventually led to its containment. Rapid deployment of field epidemiologists, establishment of treatment centers, and implementation of strict infection control measures played a crucial role in limiting the spread of the virus. Community engagement and public awareness campaigns also played a significant role in building trust and promoting adherence to preventive measures. The successful containment of the Ebola outbreak in West Africa serves as a testament to the importance of rapid response, collaboration, and innovation in managing emerging infectious diseases.

Case Study 3: COVID-19 Pandemic Response

The ongoing COVID-19 pandemic, caused by the novel coronavirus SARS-CoV-2, has highlighted both the strengths and weaknesses of global disease prevention and control efforts. Despite unprecedented measures implemented by governments and health organizations worldwide, the pandemic has resulted in millions of infections and deaths, as well as profound social and economic disruptions. However, the pandemic has also spurred remarkable scientific collaboration and innovation, leading to the rapid development and distribution of vaccines in record time. Lessons learned from the COVID-19 pandemic, including the importance of early detection, transparent communication, and equitable access to healthcare, will undoubtedly inform future strategies for managing emerging infectious diseases.

Case Study 4: HIV/AIDS Prevention and Treatment

The HIV/AIDS epidemic, which emerged in the late 20th century, represents one of the most significant public health challenges of modern times. Initially met with fear, stigma, and discrimination, the global response to HIV/AIDS has evolved over decades, leading to significant advancements in prevention, treatment, and care. Through comprehensive prevention programs, including condom distribution, needle exchange programs, and education campaigns, the spread of HIV has been successfully slowed in many regions.

Additionally, the development of antiretroviral therapy (ART) has transformed HIV infection from a death sentence to a manageable chronic condition. However, challenges remain, including access to treatment in resource-limited settings and addressing social determinants of health that contribute to HIV disparities. The response to HIV/AIDS serves as a testament to the power of community mobilization, scientific innovation, and political will in combating infectious diseases.

Case Study 5: Malaria Control and Elimination Efforts

Malaria, caused by the Plasmodium parasite and transmitted by Anopheles mosquitoes, continues to be a major global health threat, particularly in sub-Saharan Africa. However, concerted efforts by governments, international organizations, and civil society have led to significant progress in malaria control and elimination. Through initiatives such as indoor residual spraying, insecticide-treated bed nets, and prompt diagnosis and treatment, malaria incidence and mortality rates have declined in many endemic regions. Additionally, ongoing research into new tools and strategies, including novel insecticides and vaccines, holds promise for further reducing the burden of malaria. Despite these achievements, challenges remain, including drug resistance, insecticide resistance, and funding gaps. The fight against malaria underscores the importance of sustained investment, multisectoral collaboration, and innovation in disease control efforts.

Case Study 6: Tuberculosis Control and Prevention Programs

Tuberculosis (TB), caused by the bacterium Mycobacterium tuberculosis, remains a leading cause of death worldwide, particularly in low- and middle-income countries. However, through the implementation of comprehensive TB control and prevention programs, significant progress has been made in reducing TB incidence and mortality rates. Key components of these programs include early detection through improved diagnostic tools, standardized treatment regimens, and infection control measures. Additionally, efforts to address social determinants of health, such as poverty, overcrowding, and malnutrition, are critical for TB control. Despite progress, challenges such as drug-resistant TB and co-infection with HIV continue to pose significant obstacles to TB elimination efforts. The global response to TB highlights the importance of integrated, patient-centered care, as well as sustained political commitment and investment in health systems strengthening

Learning from Success

Through an analysis of these case studies, several key themes and strategies emerge:

Early Detection and Rapid Response

Timely identification of cases and swift implementation of control measures are crucial for containing outbreaks and preventing further transmission. This requires robust surveillance systems, laboratory capacity, and trained personnel to detect and respond to emerging threats quickly.

Multisectoral Collaboration

Effective disease prevention and control efforts often require collaboration across multiple sectors, including healthcare, public health, government agencies, academia, and community organizations. Coordinated action and information sharing among stakeholders are essential for mounting a comprehensive response.

Community Engagement

Engaging with affected communities is critical for building trust, promoting adherence to preventive measures, and addressing cultural, social, and economic factors that influence disease transmission. Community participation in planning, implementation, and evaluation of interventions enhances their effectiveness and sustainability.

Capacity Building

Investing in healthcare infrastructure, human resources, and technical capacity strengthens the ability of countries to detect, respond to, and recover from infectious disease outbreaks. This includes training healthcare workers, establishing laboratory networks, and improving access to essential medicines and supplies.

Innovation and Adaptation

Innovation in technologies, approaches, and interventions is essential for staying ahead of evolving pathogens and emerging threats. Research and development efforts should focus on developing new diagnostics, treatments, vaccines, and surveillance tools to improve disease prevention and control efforts.

Equity and Inclusivity

Ensuring equitable access to healthcare services, resources, and information is essential for addressing health disparities and reducing the burden of infectious diseases on vulnerable populations. Efforts to promote health equity should prioritize marginalized groups and address underlying social determinants of health.

By applying these key themes and strategies, policymakers, public health authorities, and communities can work together to strengthen disease prevention and control efforts, enhance global health security, and protect the well-being of populations worldwide. Through ongoing collaboration, innovation, and learning from past successes and challenges, we can build a safer, healthier future for all.

Chapter 8

Future Directions and Challenges

As the world grapples with the ongoing threat of emerging infectious diseases, including Alaskapox, it is crucial to consider the future trajectory of these diseases and the challenges and opportunities that lie ahead. In this chapter, we delve into the potential scenarios for the evolution and spread of Alaskapox, as well as the key challenges and opportunities for research and surveillance in mitigating its impact.

Speculations on the Future Trajectory of Alaskapox

The future trajectory of Alaskapox remains uncertain, as the virus continues to evolve and adapt within its host populations. One possible scenario is that Alaskapox may continue to spread geographically, reaching new regions beyond Alaska as a result of human encroachment into wildlife habitats and increased global connectivity. This could lead to a higher incidence of human cases and potentially greater severity of illness, particularly in vulnerable populations such as the immunocompromised.

Additionally, there is the possibility of Alaskapox undergoing genetic mutations that alter its pathogenicity or transmissibility, leading to unpredictable changes in disease dynamics. Such mutations could pose significant challenges for disease surveillance and control efforts, necessitating ongoing monitoring and adaptation of public health strategies.

Furthermore, the long-term impact of climate change on Alaskapox transmission dynamics is a subject of concern. Changes in temperature and precipitation patterns could affect the distribution and abundance of small mammal reservoirs, influencing the prevalence of the virus in wildlife populations and potentially altering patterns of human exposure.

Another factor to consider is the potential for cross-species transmission events, where Alaskapox could jump from its natural reservoir hosts to other animal species or humans. This could occur through close contact between infected and susceptible individuals, or through the introduction of the virus into new ecological niches.

In light of these uncertainties, it is essential for public health agencies and research institutions to remain vigilant and proactive in their efforts to monitor and respond to the evolving threat of Alaskapox. This includes investing in robust surveillance systems, conducting research to better understand the ecological and epidemiological factors driving disease transmission, and developing strategies for disease prevention and control.

Key Challenges and Opportunities for Research and Surveillance

The future of Alaskapox research and surveillance presents both challenges and opportunities. One of the primary challenges is the need for improved diagnostic tools and techniques to facilitate early detection of Alaskapox cases in both humans and wildlife. Current diagnostic methods rely primarily on laboratory testing, which can be time-consuming and resource-intensive. Developing rapid and reliable diagnostic assays could enhance our ability to identify and respond to outbreaks more effectively.

Another challenge is the complexity of Alaskapox transmission dynamics, which involve interactions between wildlife reservoirs, human populations, and environmental factors. Understanding these dynamics requires interdisciplinary collaboration between epidemiologists, ecologists, veterinarians, and other experts. Integrated surveillance programs that incorporate data from multiple sources, including wildlife surveys, environmental monitoring, and human health surveillance, can provide a more comprehensive understanding of Alaskapox ecology and epidemiology.

Furthermore, there is a need for research to elucidate the genetic diversity of Alaskapox strains and their implications for disease transmission and pathogenicity. By sequencing viral genomes and studying genetic variations among different strains, researchers can gain insights into the evolutionary history of the virus and identify potential targets for intervention, such as vaccine development.

Despite these challenges, there are also opportunities for innovation and progress in the field of Alaskapox research and surveillance. Advances in genomic sequencing technologies, data analytics, and computational modeling hold promise for improving our understanding of disease dynamics and informing evidence-based public health interventions.

Additionally, collaborations between academia, government agencies, and industry partners can facilitate the translation of research findings into practical solutions for disease prevention and control. By leveraging the expertise and resources of diverse stakeholders, we can enhance our collective ability to address the complex challenges posed by Alaskapox and other emerging infectious diseases.

In conclusion, the future of Alaskapox research and surveillance is marked by both uncertainty and potential. By addressing key challenges and seizing opportunities for innovation and collaboration, we can advance our understanding of the virus and develop effective strategies for mitigating its impact on human and animal health. Through sustained efforts in research, surveillance, and public health preparedness, we can work towards a future where the threat of Alaskapox is effectively managed and controlled.

CONCLUSION

In the culmination of our journey through the intricate landscape of Alaskapox and emerging infectious diseases, we find ourselves at a crossroads of knowledge and action. The story of Alaskapox serves as a poignant reminder of the complex interplay between human health, wildlife ecology, and environmental change. As we reflect on the insights gleaned from our exploration, several key themes emerge, each carrying profound implications for the future of global health security.

First and foremost, the emergence of Alaskapox underscores the urgent need for a proactive and interdisciplinary approach to disease surveillance and control. The rapid spread of Alaskapox within Alaska and its potential to impact vulnerable populations highlight the importance of early detection, timely intervention, and robust public health response strategies. By harnessing the power of collaboration between scientists, healthcare providers, policymakers, and communities, we can strengthen our capacity to detect, monitor, and mitigate the threats posed by emerging infectious diseases.

Moreover, the story of Alaskapox underscores the critical importance of understanding the ecological and environmental factors driving disease emergence and transmission. As human activities continue to encroach on natural habitats and disrupt wildlife ecosystems, the risk of zoonotic disease spillover increases.

By adopting a One Health approach that recognizes the interconnectedness of human, animal, and environmental health, we can work towards sustainable solutions that promote both ecosystem resilience and public health.

Furthermore, the societal implications of Alaskapox highlight the need for effective risk communication, community engagement, and policy interventions. By raising awareness about the potential risks posed by emerging infectious diseases and empowering individuals to take proactive measures to protect themselves and their communities, we can build resilience against future outbreaks. Additionally, by advocating for evidence-based policies that prioritize disease prevention, surveillance, and preparedness, we can create a more resilient and equitable healthcare system that safeguards the health and well-being of all.

As we look towards the future, it is clear that the challenges posed by emerging infectious diseases like Alaskapox are complex and multifaceted. Yet, they are not insurmountable. By embracing innovation, collaboration, and a shared commitment to global health security, we can navigate the uncertain terrain ahead with confidence and resilience. Together, we have the power to shape a healthier, more resilient world for generations to come.

In closing, the story of Alaskapox serves as both a cautionary tale and a call to action. It reminds us of the fragility of our interconnected world and the importance of remaining vigilant in the face of emerging threats. Yet, it also inspires us with the promise of scientific discovery, the resilience of human spirit, and the boundless potential for positive change. As we embark on the next chapter of our journey, let us do so with hope, determination, and a shared commitment to building a healthier, more sustainable future for all. With each step forward, let us remember the lessons learned from Alaskapox and strive to create a world where health, equity, and resilience are cherished values upheld by all.